THE GOUT DIET RECIPES

COOKBOOK

FOR

NEWBIES AND BEGINNERS

BY

Dr. Christen Zimmermann

Table of Contents

INTRODUCTION

Gout, a type of arthritis, can cause sudden, painful attacks. In addition to managing your weight and taking medicine, eating a healthy diet and avoiding certain foods can help prevent gout flares and ease symptoms of the condition when they occur.

Gout is a type of arthritis that occurs when uric acid crystals build up in joints, such as the big toe, wrist or knee. Purines-compounds found in your cells and some foods-are broken down into uric acid in the body. Uric acid is then excreted in the urine via the kidneys. If you produce too much uric acid or your kidneys can't efficiently remove it, the levels can become too high and lead to deposits of needle-like crystals in joints. These deposits cause pain, redness, swelling and inflammation.

Risk Factors

About 4 percent of adults in the United States have gout, and more men have it than women. The following factors can increase your risk of developing gout:

* Genetics-you are more likely to get gout if someone in your family has it.

* Obesity

* Drinking alcohol, especially beer

* Eating meats and seafood high in purines (e.g. wild game, organ meat, shellfish)

* Consuming high-fructose corn syrup

How Can Diet Affect Gout?

Purines naturally occur in red meat, seafood and some vegetables. For decades, health care professionals thought people with gout should avoid all foods high in purines. That's not the case anymore. You can say goodbye to long lists of eat-this-and-not-that foods. New research shows that not all high-purine foods must be nixed to control gout.

It is common for people with gout to have other conditions that are a part of "metabolic syndrome"-high blood pressure, high blood sugar, high cholesterol or triglycerides, and excess body fat around the waist. Therefore, a gout diet now looks very similar to a heart-healthy diet. A focus on vegetables, nuts, legumes, whole grains and fatty fish like salmon will not only prevent gout flares but will also keep you at a healthy weight and protect your heart.

Who Should Follow a Gout Diet?

If you get diagnosed with gout, your doctor will prescribe medication and lifestyle changes to help control uric acid levels. You should follow the gout diet long-term to reduce flare-ups from gout.

What's Allowed on a Gout Diet?

The gout diet is no longer about all of the foods you can't have. Research shows that some foods, such as dairy products, may actually help reduce the number of gout flares. "It is important to include a variety of fruits, vegetables, whole grains and beans or legumes into your diet," says Molly Cleary, R.D., dietitian at New York Presbyterian Hospital. "Even vegetables high in purines, which did not used to be recommended, should be safe to consume with gout," she says.

The American Association of Family Physicians (AAFP) also recommends eating vegetables, as well as consuming low-fat dairy products.

Foods You Can Eat

* Fruits

* Vegetables

* Whole grains

* Beans/legumes

* Nuts

* Some seafood

* Poultry

* Eggs

* Soy

* Low-fat dairy products

What's Not Allowed on a Gout Diet?

"No foods need to be avoided altogether, but there are certain foods that should only be consumed in limited portions," Cleary says. "Limiting organ meats and certain types of seafood-anchovies, tuna, sardines, haddock and more-may help to decrease gout attacks. Other types of seafood, including salmon, shrimp and lobster, are lower in purines and should be fine in moderate amounts. Red meat and poultry should be limited to no more than 6 ounces per day."

The cardiovascular benefits from eating heart-healthy fish like salmon and tuna might outweigh the rise in uric acid they cause. Cleary recommends replacing the protein you would be getting from meat "with nuts and nut butters, eggs, low-fat dairy, beans and soy-based products." It is safe to eat up to two daily servings of low-fat dairy.

The AAFP suggests restricting fruit juices and soft drinks with high-fructose corn syrup. Fructose can increase uric acid production. Refined carbohydrates should also be limited.

Finally, pay attention to the booze. "Alcohol can also increase uric acid production, so alcohol consumption should be limited as much as possible," Cleary says. According to a 2016 review in The American Journal of Medicine, wine is OK in moderation, but li�uor and beer should be avoided as much as possible.

Foods to Limit

* Purine-rich meat and seafood (organ meats, shellfish, salmon, sardines, tuna, herring)

* Alcohol (especially beer and li�uor)

* Beverages sweetened with high-fructose corn syrup

*Refined carbohydrates (including sugar)

Some foods and lifestyle factors may reduce your risk of getting gout and help manage gout flares if they occur.

* Vitamin C: Vitamin C may help reduce uric acid levels. Talk to your doctor and ask if you should take a vitamin C supplement.

* Weight loss: "Gout is often associated with obesity, diabetes and kidney disease," Cleary says. "Therefore, it is important to achieve and maintain a healthy weight and follow dietary guidelines related to these conditions. Weight loss can also relieve stress on the joints."

* Water: Drinking water can reduce the number of gout flares. Water helps flush uric acid our of your body.

* Cherries: Eating cherries could reduce the number of gout attacks. In a 2012 study, participants who ate cherries over the course of two days had a 35 percent lower risk of gout flares following cherry intake than those who ate no cherries. Cherries might help gout flares by reducing uric acid levels.

* Coffee: Drinking six or more cups of coffee per day is associated with a 59 percent reduced risk of getting gout.

Gout Safe Vegetable Soup

A comforting safe for gout / vegan soup loaded with fresh vegetables and red beans for protein.

Ingredients

- Homemade Vegetarian Broth
- 1 Tablespoon Oil
- 2 each leeks
- 2 each carrots
- 2 ribs celery I used four tops with leaves
- 1/4 teaspoon salt
- 8 Cups water

Soup

- 1 Tablespoon Oil
- 2 Cups Potatoes Diced
- 1 Cup Carrot Diced

• 1 Tablespoon Garlic Minced

• 1.5 Cups Red Beans cooked

• 2 sprigs Rosemary

• 4 sprigs Thyme

• 2 Cups Spinach.

Instructions

Homemade Vegetarian Broth

• To a pot on medium heat add one Tablespoon of oil and two leeks that have been cut up. Cook for about three minutes until they start to soften up.

• Add two carrots that have been cut up. Add the top of a few celery stalks with leaves. Cover with water, add 1/4 teaspoon of salt. Bring to a simmer and cook until the carrots are very tender but not �uite mush. Then turn off the heat and let it cool down a little.

• When the broth has cool to a safe to handle temperature strain out the veggies. Remove the carrots and set aside.

Then s⍰ueeze most of the li⍰uid out of the leeks and celery.

Soup

- Add the carrots to some of the broth and blend. With a pot on medium heat add one tablespoon of oil the onions, raw carrots, celery and garlic. Cook until the onions are translucent (approximately three to five minutes).

- When the onions are translucent add the broth, potatoes and the herbs. Bring to a simmer and cook ten minutes.

- Add the cauliflower and red beans. Simmer another five minutes. Add the package of frozen green beans and cook until the potatoes and cauliflower are tender (approximately another five minutes).

- At the end of cooking add two cups of spinach.

One Pot Chicken and Lentil Stew

This one pot chicken and lentil stew recipe is a light and healthy one pot meal that's bursting with creamy and zesty deliciousness! The chicken is marinated with a variety of healthy, anti-inflammatory spices, yogurt and tangy orange juice for a mouthwatering healthy meal that the whole family will love!

Ingredients

- 1 cup dried green or brown lentils
- 2 medium raw chicken breasts, cut into 1 inch cubes (thawed chicken breasts work great as well!)
- 1 tsp celery seed, divided
- 1 tsp coriander, divided
- 2 tsp paprika, divide
- 1 tsp Italian seasoning
- 1 5.3 oz container of plain Greek yogurt, reserving a few tbsp to dollop on top at the end (a little under 1 cup)
- the juice of 1/2 of a small orange, about 1/4 cup

- 1 tbsp extra virgin olive oil
- 1 red onion, peeled and sliced thin (or yellow/white onion, whatever you have)
- 1 cup coconut milk
- 2 1/2 cups chicken broth
- 1/4 tsp salt
- pinch of pepper
- parsley or cilantro as garnish

Instructions

- MAKE THE CHICKEN MARINADE – In a bowl, mix together the yogurt (reserve a couple teaspoons) 1/2 tsp celery seed, 1/2 tsp coriander, 1 tsp paprika, 1 tsp Italian seasoning and orange juice. Toss the cubed chicken with the yogurt marinade. Place in an airtight container in the refrigerator for at least 30 minutes, or overnight.
- SEAR THE CHICKEN – Heat one tbsp of olive oil over medium heat in a large cast iron dutch oven or pot with a lid. Add the marinated chicken to the pot and cook undisturbed for about 5 minutes. Toss in your chopped

red onion, flip the chicken and continue to cook for another 5 minutes, undisturbed.

- SIMMER WITH THE LENTILS – Add the green lentils, coconut milk, chicken broth, 1/2 tsp coriander, 1 tsp paprika, 1/2 tsp celery seed and salt/pepper. Stir to fully combine, place the lid on the pot and simmer for about 35 minutes, stirring occasionally to prevent sticking

- PLATE & GARNISH – Test the lentils to make sure they are not too hard. They should be soft but not mushy. Plate the lentils and chicken in a bowl. Garnish with parsley and a dollop of plain Greek yogurt and enjoy!

Chicken Broccoli Casserole with Cherries and Almonds

Chicken Broccoli Casserole with Cherries and Almonds - a healthy and delicious twist on your typical broccoli cheese casserole recipe! With shredded chicken, tender broccoli, Greek yogurt, Feta cheese, tart cherries and toasted almonds, it's a totally unexpected yet award-winning combination that's fabulously delicious!

Ingredients

1 large head of broccoli cut into bite-size florets (or buy a large bag of broccoli florets)

3 tablespoons olive oil

1 teaspoon salt

1 teaspoon pepper

3 cloves garlic, minced

⅓ cup chicken stock (use more if your think your mixture seems dry)

2 chicken breasts cooked and shredded (I used a rotisserie chicken!)

1 cup plain Greek yogurt

6 ounces Feta cheese

4 green onions, chopped

⅓ cup sliced almonds, toasted

½ cup dried tart cherries

Instructions

• Preheat oven to 425F.

• Clean and cut broccoli florets into bite-sized pieces, drizzle with olive oil, and sprinkle with salt and pepper. Bake in a 9 X 13 baking dish for 10 minutes at 425 degrees. While the broccoli is roasting, shred the chicken and set it aside.

• Heat up a medium-sized skillet on the stove, add olive oil and minced garlic. Cook for 1 minute then add the chicken stock, and bring to a simmer. Add the chicken and stir. Fold in the Greek yogurt, 3 ounces of the feta cheese, green onions, half the cherries and half the almonds.

• When the broccoli is finished roasting, turn the oven temp down to 375, and fold the chicken mixture into the baking dish with the broccoli. Then sprinkle with the remaining feta, almonds and cherries.

• Bake for 15-20 minutes covered, and serve.

Superfoods Salad

We will feel younger, healthier, energetic and less moody when we feed our body with an amazing selection of fresh and colorful food, such as this amazing salad.

Ingredients

• 4 cups Fresh Kale

• 1 1/2 cup Shredded Carrots

• 1 1/2 cup Broccoli Slaw

• 1 1/2 cup Mukimame or deshelled Edamame

• 1 1/2 cup Blueberry

• 64 Cashews 16 per serving

• 1 cup Walnuts 12 to 14 halves per serving

• 1/4 cup hulled Sunflower Seeds

• 1/2 cup Dried Cranberry

Lemon-Ginger Vinaigrette

• 1 large Ripe Lemon s⍰ueeze as much as you can (if the lemon is smaller, you can use 2)

• 1/4 cup Olive Oil

• 3 tbsp. Apple Cider Vinegar or red wine vinegar

• 1 inch Fresh Ginger grated

• 1 teaspoon minced Garlic

• 1 teaspoon Dried Parsley

• 1/4 teaspoon Chili Powder

• Himalayan Salt to taste

Instructions

1. Wash all the vegetables and fruit, then prepare them by slicing, shredding, and grating.

2. Slice Kale into bite size pieces, and place in the large bowl.

3. Mix everything for lemon-ginger vinaigrette in the glass jar with a fitted lid and season with salt to taste, start with 1/4 teaspoon and taste. Close the lid and shake the jar to combine all the ingredients.

4. Pour the vinaigrette over the kale and massage it for about one minute or until the kale is tender. S□ueeze the

kale using your hands. You will end up with half of the size in the bowl. You got to do this step to make kale tastier.

5. Now add all the other ingredients (fruits and vegetables) and lightly toss with the kale.

6. Taste and see if you need to add a pinch or two of Salt.

7. Serve just a salad immediately or place in the container/jar with a fitted lid and keep in the fridge for up to 2 days.

Potato Leek Soup

Ingredients

- 3 tablespoons unsalted grass-fed butter, ghee or coconut oil
- 4 washed leeks, white AND green parts, roughly chopped
- 3 cloves garlic, peeled and smashed
- ¾ cup of cooking sherry
- 2 lbs yukon or russet potatoes, (cauliflower for paleo) scrubbed/washed well and roughly chopped into ½-inch pieces
- 8 cups bone broth or chicken stock or veggie stock
- 2 bay leaves
- 1½ teaspoons finely chopped fresh thyme
- 1 teaspoon sea salt
- ¼ teaspoon ground black pepper
- 1 cup plain cashew cream

- 2 tablespoons Braggs (with the mother!) apple cider vinegar
- ¾ cup of nutritional yeast (great source of protein)
- Chives, finely chopped (optional)
- Bacon, chopped in small cubes (optional)
- Grated asiago cheese (optional)
- Chili Oil (optional for drizzling)

Instructions

- Melt the butter over medium heat in a large dutch oven. (Just my preference for making soups.) Add the leeks and garlic and to simmer, stirring regularly, until soft and wilted, about 10 minutes. No browning allowed, but sherry splashing to deglaze encouraged.
- Add the potatoes (or separately steamed and drained cauliflower), stock/broth of choice, bay leaves, thyme, salt and pepper to pot and bring to a slow boil. Cover and turn the heat down to low.
- Simmer for 20 minutes, or until the potatoes are very soft and break apart when smooshed with a fork. If using

cauliflower you can immediately blend after adding it COOKED into the broth mixture.

• Fish out bay leaves, then add the nutritional yeast and purée the soup with a hand-held immersion blender until smooth.

• Add the cashew cream and apple cider vinegar and bring to a simmer. Taste and adjust seasoning with salt and pepper. Garnish whichever way you like!

Cherry Walnut Smoothie

Cherry walnut smoothies are packed with antioxidants and make for a well-balanced breakfast.

Ingredients

- 1 ripe banana, peeled and frozen
- 1 cup ripe cherries, pitted
- 3/4 cup unsweetened almond milk
- 2 tablespoons full fat coconut milk
- 2 tablespoons raw walnuts, chopped

Instructions

1. Put it all in a blender and blend until smooth.

Vegan Cajun Red Quinoa and Rice

Slow-cooked red beans is the secret to these amazing cajun dish. They really soak up the flavor and have the most incredible texture that you just can't get from canned beans. Wonderful, deep cajun spices and heat make this dish addicting and is also super filling from the �uinoa and beans.

Ingredients

- For the Beans
- 1 lb bag of dry red kidney beans Making them from scratch yields fabulous tasting beans! Do not skimp on these!
- 2 teaspoons of garlic powder
- 2 teaspoons of paprika
- 1 teaspoon onion powder
- 1 1/2 teaspoons of sea salt
- For the Quinoa

• 1 cup red quinoa not white! my recipe is specific to use the red quinoa for texture

• 2 cups low-sodium vegetable broth

• 2 small bay leaves

• 1/2 teaspoon garlic powder

• 1/2 teaspoon paprika

• 1/2 teaspoon fine sea salt

• 1 teaspoon Cajun seasoning

• 1/4 teaspoon thyme leaves

• 1/4 teaspoon smoked paprika

• 1/4 teaspoon ground chipotle chili spice or red pepper or cayenne pepper

• Few grinds of fresh ground black pepper

• Veggies

• 1 large green bell pepper chopped

• 1/2 large red onion chopped (130 g, about a cup)

• 3 large garlic cloves minced

• salt & pepper

Instructions

1. Ahead of time prepare the red beans according to package directions either overnight or early in the day. I went ahead and used the whole bag just to have extra beans, but you will not need all of them at the time of this recipe. This will need to be done in advance prior to making the quinoa and veggies. Once you have already done the soak method of the beans, you can then cook them. Follow the cooking directions on the back of the bag.

2. Prepare the quinoa. Add the quinoa, vegetable broth and all the spices, including the bay leaves, into a pot. Bring to a boil. Once boiling, cover and turn heat to low and cook for 20-25 minutes or until almost all of the water has evaporated, stirring a few times during the cooking process. Once the water is almost gone, turn the heat off, return the lid and leave covered for 5 minutes. Remove the lid and fluff with a fork.

3. While the □uinoa is cooking, prepare the vegetables. Pour a few tablespoons of broth in a large pan and turn

the heat to medium low. Add the bell pepper and onion into a large pan. Add some salt and pepper. Once they are almost tender, after 5-10 minutes, add the garlic and cook until all veggies are tender stirring often so the garlic doesn't burn. Add more broth if necessary. Turn the heat off. Combine the veggies and quinoa.

4. Serve by plating with the quinoa mixture and adding the cooked beans on top. Season with extra salt or cajun spice if desired.

Healthy Lemon Garlic Salmon

This Healthy Lemon Garlic Salmon is easy to make and ready in under 15 minutes. It's healthy, low calorie, and only uses a handful of ingredients!

Ingredients

• 4 salmon portions skin-on

• 1/2 teaspoon salt

• 1/2 teaspoon black pepper

• 2 teaspoons extra virgin olive oil

• 4 tablespoons fresh lemon juice

• 8 garlic cloves crushed

• 2 tablespoons finely chopped fresh dill

Instructions

1. Season salmon portions with salt and pepper.

2. Heat a large heavy skillet over medium-high heat. Add in olive oil and heat 30 seconds. Place salmon portions into the skillet, starting with the skin side up. Sear 3 to 4

minutes, then flip over and sear the other side 3 more minutes. Move salmon to one side of the pan.

3. Pour lemon juice into empty area of skillet and in garlic cloves and saute 60 seconds. Spoon garlic lemon juice over salmon and cook until fish is cooked through and flakes easily with a fork.

4. Sprinkle fresh dill on top of salmon portions and serve immediately. Garnish with lemon slices if desired.

Sweet Potato Turmeric Soup

This detox sweet potato turmeric soup is healthy in the best kind of way. It's chock-full of naturally anti-inflammatory and flavourful ingredients like turmeric, ginger, and garlic, and made creamy with almond butter and coconut milk. It's a warming, feel-good soup for cooler-weather days, or anytime your body's craving something easy to digest. It's simple to make and reheat, and is ready in under 30 minutes!

Ingredients

• 1 tablespoon coconut oil

• 1 medium onion, chopped

• ¼ cup chopped ginger

• 4 cloves garlic, peeled and smashed with the side of your knife

• 1 large sweet potato, peeled and diced (about 1.5 lbs)

• 2 large carrots, chopped

• 1 tablespoon EACH: turmeric and sea salt

• ½ teaspoon EACH: black pepper and cayenne pepper

- 4 cups chicken stock, or beef bone broth
- 6 tablespoons almond butter
- 15 ounce can coconut milk
- Juice from one lime
- Minced cilantro, to serve
- Salty Almond Croutons
- 1 teaspoon coconut oil
- ½ cup chopped almonds
- 1 tablespoon soy sauce, can sub gluten-free or coco aminos

Instructions

- Add the coconut oil to a large pot over medium-high heat. When it melts, add the onion and let it cook for 3-4 minutes. Add the garlic and ginger and cook for 1 more minute. Mix in the sweet potato, carrots, turmeric (see notes), sea salt, black pepper, and cayenne.

• Add the stock to the pot and bring the pot to a boil. Reduce the heat to medium and simmer, partially covered, for 10 minutes, or until the vegetables are soft.

• Make the almond croutons while the soup cooks. Heat the coconut oil in a small pan over medium-high heat. Add the chopped almonds and toast until fragrant and golden, about 5 minutes, shaking the pan a few times. Add the soy sauce to the pan and let it boil until it's gone and the almonds are coated. Remove the pan from the heat.

• Transfer the soup to your blender, add the almond butter, and blend until smooth.

• Pour the soup back into the pot, add the coconut milk and lime juice. Season to taste with salt and heat through. Serve the turmeric soup topped with salty almond croutons and a little minced cilantro.

Cherry Chia Greek Yogurt Bowls

Packed with antioxidant-rich cherries, this yogurt bowl is ideal after a tough workout for pain relief and recovery.

Ingredients

Chia Seed Jam

- 2 cups Chelan Fresh Sweet Cherries pitted
- 3 tbsp chia seeds
- 2 tbsp honey
- 1/4 cup water

For Each Greek Yogurt Bowl

- 1 cup nonfat plain greek yogurt
- 1/2 tsp vanilla extract
- 1 tsp hemp seeds
- 1 tbsp granola

Instructions

To Make Chia Seed Jam:

1. Add cherries, chia seeds, honey, and water to a small pot on high. Using a potato masher, mash down cherries and stir to combine with the other ingredients. Bring to a boil, then turn down the heat and let simmer for 10 minutes stirring constantly.

To Make Greek Yogurt Bowls

1. Mix greek yogurt with vanilla extract. Top greek yogurt with 2 tablespoons cherry chia seed jam, hemp hearts, granola, and a few additional Chelan Fresh Sweet Cherries. Eat within one hour of working out.

Chicken and Vegetable Fried rice

This healthy chicken and vegetables fried rice recipe is loaded with vegetables and made with whole grain brown rice. This kid-friendly family favorite is also naturally gluten-free!

Ingredients

- 8 oz chicken breast (diced)
- 1 medium onion (diced)
- 1 medium zucchini (diced)
- 1 ear corn (kernels removed)
- 1 c green peas
- ½ c edamame (shelled and cooked)
- 2 c broccoli (cooked and cut into small florets)
- 1 egg
- 2 c leftover brown rice (preferably cold)
- 1 tbs sesame oil
- 2 tbs soy sauce (low sodium)

• 1 tbs rice wine vinegar

• 1 c scallions (minced)

Instructions

• Heat a wok or large pan over medium-high heat and spray with non-stick spray.(Tip: Save the sesame oil calories to finish the dish vs. using them to cook the ingredients. You won't miss the calories and you won't notice a change in flavor.)

• Saute chicken breast about 4 minutes per side. No need to move the chicken constantly – let it brown and gain flavor.

• Once cooked, remove from pan and reserve. In the same pan, add onion and zucchini; cook for 3-4 minutes. Add corn kernels, peas, edamame and broccoli. Stir fry for about 2 minutes to heat.

• Move the veggies to the perimeter of the pan and in the middle, add the egg. Using a wooden spoon, quickly stir the egg to scramble. Add the reserved, cold brown rice, cooked chicken and sesame oil. Stir well to distribute the oil and spread the rice and veggies all over the pan.

• Walk away from the pan and let the ingredients brown a bit. After about 2 minutes, stir and let sit for another 2 minutes to brown. Add soy sauce, rice vinegar and scallions. Stir well and serve.

Vegetable Jambalaya

This easy Vegetable Jambalaya has amazing flavor with a bit of spice. I've got simple tips for creating satisfying vegetarian dishes to make all the difference!

Ingredients

- 1/4 cup extra-virgin olive oil
- 1 medium sweet onion sliced
- 2 stalks celery cut into 1/2-inch slices
- 2 medium carrots cut into 1/2-inch slices
- 1 medium red bell pepper sliced
- 3 to 4 cloves garlic minced
- 1 teaspoon hot smoked paprika
- 1/8 teaspoon ground cayenne pepper
- 2 teaspoons dried oregano
- 1 teaspoon dried thyme leaves
- 2 bay leaves
- Kosher salt

- freshly ground black pepper
- 15- ounce can diced fire-roasted tomatoes
- 1 1/4 cups white rice
- 2 1/2 cups vegetable broth
- 15- ounce can black-eyed peas drained and rinsed
- 8- ounces frozen cut okra
- hot pepper sauce
- handful chopped celery leaves or fresh parsley

Instructions

- Heat the olive oil in a 10-inch skillet or braiser over medium-high heat. Add the onion, celery and carrots. Cook, stirring fre�uently, for about 6 minutes or until the onions become a bit soft. Add the red pepper and continue to cook for about 3 minutes. Add the garlic, paprika, cayenne, oregano, thyme, bay leaves, salt and pepper. Stir to coat and add the tomatoes. Cook for 2 minutes. Add the rice. Stir to coat. Add the vegetable broth and stir

• Cover the pot, increase the heat a bit and bring to a boil. Immediately reduce the heat to a simmer. Cook the rice covered for 10 minutes. Add the black-eyed peas and okra just over the top of the rice and cover. Cook for an additional 10 to 15 minutes or until the okra is tender and the rice is cooked. Remove from the heat, keeping the pot covered and allow it to sit for 5 minutes before serving.

• Stir and fluff the rice with a large fork. Top with your favorite hot sauce and a handful of chopped celery leaves or parsley.

Tart Cherry Sorbet

Tart Cherry Sorbet: made with tart cherries and fresh orange, a refreshing treat on a hot summer night

Ingredients

- 4 cups pitted tart cherries
- 6 tbsp agave nectar, date paste, honey, or maple syrup (agave & date paste are more neutral tasting), or less is using sweet cherries
- 1½ tsp fresh orange zest (about ½ the orange)
- 1½ tbsp fresh orange juice
- ⅛-1/4 tsp ground black pepper
- pinch of fresh ground nutmeg

Instructions

1. Place all ingredients into a high-speed blender, like a Vitamix.

2. Add to an ice cream maker, and process until sorbet thickens.

3. Remove from ice cream maker, and place into a freezer-safe container to harden

4. Serve in scoops alongside a

5. Chocolate ganache torte, or on top of my orange coconut tartlets.

6. To assemble tartlets, use a small ice cream scoop or melon baller and place on top of frozen tartlet shells. Refreeze together until ready to serve. Do assembly day of serving, but each part can be made ahead.

Vegan Sweet Potato Shepherd's Pie

Vegan Sweet Potato Shepherd's Pie! Packed with beans, vegetables, amazing spices and topped with mashed sweet potatoes. Healthy, hearty, delicious and something even your flesh-eating friends will enjoy.

Ingredients

- 5 medium to large sweet potatoes
- 2 stalks of celery, chopped
- 2 carrots, chopped
- 1 red onion, sliced
- 3 cloves of garlic, minced
- 1 Tbsp ground coriander
- 1 tsp. dried parsley
- 1 tsp. dried thyme
- 1 tsp. dried rosemary
- 8 oz. chopped mushrooms (I prefer cremini or baby bellas)

• 8 sun-dried tomatoes (NOT PACKED IN OIL, I prefer Trader Joe's brand)

• ½ cup low-sodium vegetable stock

• 1 x 15-ounce can of lentils or 2 cups cooked lentils. (if canned, use low-sodium or no salt added. Be sure to drain and rinse)

• 1 x 15-ounce can of chickpeas drained and rinsed (use low-sodium or no salt added)

• Salt and pepper to taste

Instructions

• Preheat oven to 425 degrees.

• Prick sweet potatoes all over with a fork, place on baking pan, and cook for 30 minutes or until they tender enough to mash with a fork. Once the sweet potatoes are done, remove from the oven, mash with skins on, and set aside.

• Reset oven to 350 degrees for later on in the recipe.

• Preheat large nonstick pan over medium-high heat. When pan is ready add celery and carrots. Let cook for 2-3 minutes adding a little veggie broth if necessary to prevent sticking. Toss in the onions and let cook for another 1-2 minutes. Add the garlic, coriander, parsley, thyme and rosemary along with 1-2 Tbsp. of veggie stock. Allow to cook for 5-10 minutes.

• While mixture cooks, slice mushrooms and chop up the sun-dried tomatoes. (If you bought sliced mushrooms just chill for a few minutes.) Add the mushrooms, sun-dried tomatoes, and veggie stock. Let cook for about 10 minutes.

• Add the lentils and chickpeas. Mix well to combine. Taste and season with salt and pepper if desired.

• Once everything is mixed together pour into a 9×11 or 9×13 baking dish (affiliate link), spread the mashed sweet potatoes evenly over mixture. Put back in oven and bake for 10 minutes allowing the whole dish to get hot.

• Remove from oven and enjoy!

Chargrilled French Beans with Chili & Garlic

These flavorful, spicy beans make for a delectable side dish, or served with a heaping scoop of □uinoa for a veggie-packed meal all on its own.

Ingredients

• 500 gm (1 lb) French beans, washed & trimmed

• 3 T. extra-virgin olive oil

• 4 garlic cloves, thinly sliced

• 2 long red (mild) chilies, thinly sliced (remove seeds if you want it really mild)

• coarse salt & freshly ground black pepper

• lemon zest to serve

Instructions

• In a large pot of boiling water, blanch the beans for 90 seconds. Transfer immediately to a bowl of ice water to stop the cooking. Drain, then dry in a kitchen towel. Toss the beans with 1/2 T. of the olive oil.

• Heat a griddle pan (or skillet) over high heat. Grill the beans in batches for about 5 minutes or until they have grill marks. Transfer grilled beans to a serving plate.

• Meanwhile, in a small saucepan, heat the rest of the olive oil (2 1/2 T.) over low heat with the chilies and garlic. Watch carefully and remove from the heat just when the garlic begins to turn golden- it will keep getting darker even off the flame.

• Pour garlic/chili oil over the grilled beans. Season with salt & pepper & the lemon zest. Makes 4 large servings.

Vegetarian Black Bean Enchilada Casserole

Simple ingredients with brilliant flavor and a little heat make this vegetarian dish a must.

Ingredients

- 24-28 corn tortillas
- 3 ½ cups red enchilada sauce
- 1 tablespoon El Pato or your favorite Jalapeño sauce
- 1 red bell pepper, diced
- 1 green bell pepper diced
- 1 ½ cups sweet yellow corn kernels, cooked
- 2 15 oz can black beans, rinsed and drained
- 2 cups shredded cheddar cheese and monterey jack cheese blend
- Fresh cilantro, diced for garnish
- Green onion, thinly sliced for garnish

Instructions

1. Preheat oven to 375°F. Grease a 9X13 casserole dish and set aside.

2. Combine enchilada sauce and El Pato in a bowl until fully mixed.

3. Spread about ½ a cup on the bottom of the pan.

4. Lay 6-8 tortillas on the bottom of the pan (overlapping is fine).

5. Spread about 1 cup of the mixed sauce onto the tortillas, fully coating them.

6. Sprinkle half the beans, half the corn, and half of the bell pepper on top of the sauced tortillas and top with a third of the cheese blend.

7. Repeat the layering process starting again with the tortillas, then add sauce, then the rest of the beans, bell pepper, corn, and another third of the cheese.

8. Top this second layer with another 8 tortillas. Coat with the remaining sauce and sprinkle the rest of the cheese on top.

9. Place in the middle rack of the oven for 45 - 55 minutes, until the sauce is bubbling, cheese is melted and the middle is cooked through.

10. Let cool for about 5 minutes. Sprinkle with fresh cilantro and serve immediately.

Italian Chicken Casserole

This is a recipe for a creamy baked chicken spaghetti recipe. It doesn't contain any "cream of" soups and it's very simple to make.

Ingredients

• 2 tablespoons olive oil

• 1 cup onion, chopped

• 3 garlic cloves, minced

• 3 cups chicken, cooked and chopped

• 2 (14 1/2 ounce) cans diced tomatoes with garlic, basil and oregano

• 1 cup heavy whipping cream

• 1 (3 ounce) package cream cheese, softened

• 2 cups mozzarella cheese, shredded

• 1 (8 ounce) package angel hair pasta, cooked and kept warm

Directions

• Preheat oven to 350 degrees; lightly spray a 9x13-inch baking dish with nonstick spray.

• In large skillet, heat olive oil over medium-high heat.

• Add onion and garlic; cook 3 minutes, or until tender.

• Stir in chicken, tomatoes and cream.

• Bring to a boil over medium-high heat; reduce heat, and simmer 10 minutes, or until slightly thickened.

• Add cream cheese and 1 cup mozzarella cheese; cook, stirring constantly until cheeses are melted.

• Add pasta, tossing gently to coat.

• Spoon into prepared baking dish.

• Sprinkle evenly with remaining cheese.

• Bake 30 minutes.

Baked Spinach and Ricotta Meatballs

Baked Spinach and Ricotta Meatballs are easy to make and will be a family favorite! Perfect addition to Sunday Supper!

Ingredients:

- 1.25 lean ground beef
- 1/2 cup part-skim ricotta
- 2 handfuls fresh spinach leaves, sliced thin
- 1/2 tsp garlic powder
- 1/2 tsp onion powder
- 1/2 teaspoon kosher salt
- fresh ground pepper, pinch
- 2 eggs, whisked
- 1/2 cup whole wheat panko
- 1/4 cup grated Parmesan
- 1 tablespoon oil
- 2 cups prepared marinara sauce

• mozzarella cheese

Directions:

1. Preheat oven to 375 degrees.

2. In a large mixing bowl, gently mix together ground beef, ricotta, spinach, garlic powder, onion powder, salt, pepper, eggs, panko and Parmesan cheese. I use my hands to combine (it helps to spread the ingredients better without over mixing).

3. Heat your large oven proof pan over medium-high heat. Add 1 tablespoon cooking oil to pan (tilt pan to spread oil around). Roll meatballs (into slightly bigger than golf ball size) and carefully add to pan. Let meatballs sear for 2-3 minutes on each side until outside of meatballs is browned. Use tongs to turn meatballs in pan. Make sure to let the side searing get a good cook on it before turning (to keep from sticking and falling apart).

4. Turn off heat. Add marinara sauce to pan, covering all of your meatballs with sauce. Cover pan with lid and place in oven and bake for 20 minutes until sauce is bubbling. Add mozzarella cheese to meatballs and bake uncovered for another 5-10 minutes until cheese is melted.

5. Serve meatballs on their own, in rolls, with whole wheat pasta, over polenta or over sauteed kale. Enjoy!

Spinach And Ricotta Stuffed Peppers

This low carb version of one of my favorite spinach and ricotta stuffed shells recipe makes weeknight dinners a breeze

Ingredients

- 1/2 cup cherry tomatoes
- 1 1/2 tablespoons olive oil
- kosher salt, to taste
- black pepper to taste
- 4 bell peppers, sliced in half lengthwise
- 2 cups spinach
- 4 cloves of garlic, minced
- 1/2 yellow onion, chopped
- 25 ounces ricotta cheese, drained*
- 1/2 tablespoon red pepper flakes
- 1 egg
- 2 tablespoons fresh chopped basil

• 1 lemon, zest

• parmesan cheese, to taste

Instructions

1. Preheat oven to 375 F.

2. Add cherry tomatoes, 1/2 tablespoon olive oil, salt, and pepper to a 9 x 11 inch oven safe baking dish. Toss them in the pan to combine. Place peppers in the pan and bake for 10 minutes.

3. While the tomatoes and peppers are cooking, heat 1 tbsp of olive oil over medium-high heat and sauté spinach, garlic, and onions until spinach has wilted. Drain the spinach well (I like to use a fine mesh strainer) and set aside in a mixing bowl.

4. Add ricotta, red pepper flakes, egg, basil, and lemon zest to the mixing bowl with the spinach and mix until fully combined.

5. Remove the peppers from the oven and stuff with the spinach and ricotta mixture. Top each pepper with about half a tablespoon of shredded parmesan cheese.

6. Place the stuffed peppers in the oven and bake for about 5 minutes, just until the cheese on top has melted and the peppers are warm all the way through. Don't bake them too long or they will become watery inside!

Lemon Garlic Pasta with Fresh Veggies

This pasta dish is a great source of vitamins and minerals so eat up and be happy.

Ingredients

• 2 cups whole-wheat fusilli high protein (such as Barilla Plus) or penne (or other short pasta) for substitute, uncooked

• 2 tablespoons extra virgin olive oil

• 2 cups broccoli florets

• 1/4 cup red onions diced

• 1 red bell pepper stemmed, seeded, and sliced into strips

• 1 zucchini small to medium, cut in half lengthwise and sliced

• 2 garlic cloves peeled and sliced

• 1/2 cup chicken broth or vegetable broth, low-sodium

• 1 cup cherry tomatoes halved

• 1/2 cup basil leaves fresh, torn into pieces and loosely packed

• 1 tablespoon lemon juice freshly s�ueezed

• 1/2 teaspoon kosher or sea salt divided

• 1/4 teaspoon black pepper

• 1/4 teaspoon red pepper flakes

Instructions

1. Cook pasta according to package directions and drain.

2. Add olive oil to a large skillet over medium heat. Add broccoli, onions, red pepper, and zucchini.

3. Sprinkle with half the salt and cook for 5 minutes, stirring occasionally, until onions are translucent.

4. Add garlic and cook for 30 seconds to 1 minute, until fragrant.

5. Add broth and tomatoes and cook for an additional 3 minutes. Toss in cooked pasta.

6. Remove from heat and toss in the torn basil leaves. Sprinkle in lemon juice, the rest of the salt, black pepper, and chili flakes. Stir to combine ingredients.

7. Enjoy!

Roasted Garlic-Parmesan Zucchini, Squash and Tomatoes

Flavor packed roasted zucchini, s□uash and tomatoes made with garlic, parmesan cheese and herbs. These sheet pan veggies are incredibly simple yet full of delicious flavor and make a great healthy, easy summer side dish to any meal.

Ingredients

• 2 small zucchini (1 lb), cut into 1/2-inch thick slices

• 2 small yellow s□uash (1 lb), cut into 1/2-inch thick slices

• 14 oz Flavorino or small Campari tomatoes , sliced into halves

• 3 Tbsp olive oil

• 4 cloves garlic , minced (1 1/2 Tbsp)

• 1 1/4 tsp Italian seasoning

• Salt and freshly ground black pepper

• 1 cup (2.4 oz) finely shredded Parmesan cheese

• Fresh or dried parsley , for garnish (optional)

Instructions

1. Preheat oven to 400 degrees. Line an 18 by 13-inch rimmed baking sheet with a sheet of parchment paper or aluminum foil.

2. In a small bowl whisk together olive oil, garlic and Italian seasoning (if possible let rest 5 - 10 minutes to allow flavors to infuse into oil). Place zucchini, squash and tomatoes in a large mixing bowl. Pour olive oil mixture over top and gently toss with hands to evenly coat.

3. Pour onto prepared baking dish and spread into an even layer. Season with salt and pepper. Sprinkle Parmesan over the top of each. Roast in preheated oven 25 - 30 minutes until veggies are tender and Parmesan is golden brown. Garnish with parsley if desired and serve warm.

Grilled Barbecue Chicken and Vegetable Foil Packs

Grilled Barbecue Chicken and Vegetables in Foil is such an easy recipe! Tender chicken covered in BBQ sauce and cooked on the grill inside foil packs!

Ingredients

- 8 aluminum foil sheets large enough to wrap around one chicken breast
- 4 (4-ounces each) boneless, skinless chicken breasts
- 1/2- cup barbecue sauce (use your favorite)
- 1 zucchini , sliced into thin rounds
- 1 red , green or yellow bell pepper, cut into thin strips
- 8 asparagus spears
- salt and fresh ground pepper , to taste
- extra virgin olive oil

Instructions

• Preheat the grill to medium-high heat. For each foil pack, prepare two sheets of aluminum foil; place the sheets one on top of the other for durability.

• Place one chicken breast on each stacked pair of foil sheets; season with salt and fresh ground pepper.

• Brush each chicken breast with 1 to 2 tablespoons barbecue sauce. Divide equally and arrange vegetables around each chicken breast; season with salt and pepper. Drizzle chicken and vegetables with little olive oil.

• Fold the sides of the foil over the chicken, covering completely; seal the packets closed. Transfer foil packets to the preheated grill rack and cook for 20 to 25 minutes, or until done, turning once.

• Chicken is done when thermometer reads 165 F. Allow the chicken to rest for a few minutes.

• Serve.

Chicken Fajita Kebabs

Chicken pieces are soaked in a bright, citrusy, well season marinade then threaded onto skewers along with fresh bell peppers and onions. Then they're grilled over hot flames to give them that fire kissed flavour we all crave! Such a fun twist on the classic chicken fajitas.

Ingredients

• 2 tsp. lime zest

• 3 Tbsp. fresh lime juice

• 3 Tbsp. orange juice (mandarin or navel)

• 3 Tbsp. olive oil, plus more for brushing grill

• 1 Tbsp. minced garlic (3 cloves)

• 1 tsp. packed brown sugar

• 2 tsp. chilli powder (preferably 1 tsp. regular 1 tsp. ancho)

• 2 tsp. ground cumin

• 2 tsp. minced canned chipotle pepper, or more to taste (about 1 pepper)

• 3 Tbsp. minced fresh cilantro, plus more for garnish

• 1 tsp. salt

• 3/4 tsp. freshly ground black pepper

• 1 3/4 lbs. boneless skinless chicken breasts, diced into 1 1/4-inch pieces

• 1 large yellow onion peeled and diced into 1-inch chunks

• 3 bell peppers (preferably 1 red, 1 yellow, 1 green), cored and diced into 1-inch pieces

Instructions

1. If using wooden skewers soak in water overnight or at least 1 hour.

2. In a mixing bowl whisk together lime zest, lime juice, orange juice, olive oil, garlic, brown sugar, chili powder, cumin, chipotle pepper, cilantro, salt and pepper.

3. Place chicken in a gallon size resealable bag then pour marinade mixture over chicken.

4. Seal bag while pressing out excess air, rub marinade over chicken and transfer to refrigerator.

5. Let marinate at least 1 hour and up to 6 hours.

6. Preheat grill over medium-high heat to 400 degrees.

7. Thread chicken and peppers onto skewers (similar to the pattern pictured).

8. Brush grill grates with oil the place skewers on grill and grill until center registers 165, about 6 minutes per side.

9. Serve warm garnished with cilantro. I recommend serving over □uinoa or cilantro lime rice or serve in warmed tortillas.

Salmon and Summer Veggies in Foil

A healthy easy salmon recipe! Individual salmon fillets are cooked in foil with zucchini, s⍰uash, tomatoes and fresh herbs. A great recipe to make in the summer to use up all those veggies.

Ingredients

• 4 (5 - 6 oz) skinless salmon fillets

• 2 small zucchini (13 oz) sliced into half moons

• 2 small yellow squash (13 oz) sliced into half moons

• 2 shallots , 1 thinly sliced and 1 chopped (there are usually two in a whole shallot)

• 1 clove garlic , minced

• 2 1/2 Tbsp olive oil , divided

• Salt and freshly ground black pepper

• 1 1/2 Tbsp fresh lemon juice

• 2 large Roma tomatoes , diced

• 1 Tbsp chopped fresh thyme (or 1 tsp dried)

- 3/4 tsp dried oregano
- 1/2 tsp dried marjoram

Instructions

1. Preheat oven to 400 degrees. Cut 4 sheets of aluminum foil into 17-inch lengths.

2. Toss zucchini, s□uash, sliced shallot and garlic together with 1 Tbsp olive oil. Season with salt and pepper to taste and divide among 4 sheets of foil, placing veggies in center of foil.

3. Brush salmon fillets with 1 Tbsp of the olive oil, season bottom side with salt and pepper then place one fillet over each layer of veggies on foil. Drizzle lemon juice over salmon and season top with salt and pepper.

4. Toss together tomatoes, remaining diced shallot, thyme, oregano and marjoram with remaining 1 1/2 tsp olive oil and season lightly with salt and pepper.

5. Divide tomato mixture over salmon fillets. Wrap sides of foil inward then fold up ends to seal.

6. Place on a rimmed baking sheet and bake in preheated oven until salmon has cooked through, about 25 - 30 minutes (cook time may vary based on thickness of salmon fillets). Carefully open foil packets and serve warm.

Italian Herb Bruschetta Chicken

Italian Herb Bruschetta Chicken is a low carb alternative to a traditional Bruschetta! Transform ordinary chicken into a delicious, flavourful meal!

Ingredients

For The Chicken:

• 2 large boneless, skinless chicken breasts halved horizontally to make 4 fillets

• 3 teaspoons Italian seasoning*

• 2 teaspoons minced garlic

• salt to taste

• 1 tablespoon of olive oil (for cooking)

For The Topping:

• 4 Roma tomatoes finely chopped

• 1/4 of a red onion finely chopped (or 3 cloves finely chopped garlic)

• 4 tablespoons shredded fresh basil

- 2 tablespoons olive oil
- salt to taste
- ½ cup freshly shaved parmesan cheese

Balsamic Glaze: (you can use store bought, or this recipe)

- 1/2 cup balsamic vinegar
- 2 teaspoons brown sugar (OPTIONAL)

Instructions

1. Season chicken with Italian seasoning, garlic and salt. Heat oil in a grill pan or skillet, and sear chicken breasts over medium-high heat until browned on both sides and cooked through (about 6 minutes each side). Remove from pan; set aside and allow to rest.

2. Combine the tomatoes, red onion, basil, olive oil in a bowl. Season with salt. Top each chicken breast with the tomato mixture and parmesan cheese.

3. Serve immediately with balsamic glaze (optional).

For The Balsamic Glaze:

1. (If making from scratch, prepare while chicken is cooking.) Combine sugar (if using) and vinegar in a small saucepan over high heat and bring to the boil. Reduce heat to low; allow to simmer for 5-8 minutes or until mixture has thickened and reduced to a glaze. (If not using sugar, allow to reduce for 12-15 minutes on low heat).

Creamy Tomato Lasagna Florentine

This Creamy Tomato Lasagna Florentine is so deliciously comforting and simple. Noodles, tomato sauce, and a creamy spinach layer!

Ingredients

- 1 tablespoon olive oil
- 2–3 cloves garlic, minced
- 4–5 cups fresh spinach
- 2 cups 4% cottage cheese
- 2 eggs
- 1/4 cup ground flaxmeal (optional,
- 1 teaspoon oregano
- 1 teaspoon Italian seasoning (mine was salty – if you're using a non-salted variety, add an additional 1/4–1/2 teaspoon salt)
- a very tiny dusting of nutmeg
- a s�ueeze of lemon juice

- 1/2 cup Parmesan cheese
- 4 cups tomato sauce
- 12 no-boil or oven ready lasagna noodles
- 3–4 cups shredded Mozzarella cheese
- Chopped fresh parsley and grated Parmesan cheese for serving

Instructions

- Preheat the oven to 350 degrees. Heat the olive oil in a medium pan over medium high heat. Add the garlic and saute for 1-2 minutes. Add the spinach and stir around until just barely wilted. Remove from heat and set aside.
- Blend the cottage cheese in a food processor or blender until mostly smooth and creamy. Transfer to a bowl and mix with eggs, flaxmeal, oregano, Italian seasoning, nutmeg, lemon juice, and Parmesan cheese. Stir in the spinach and set aside.
- To assemble lasagna, spray a 9×13 baking dish with nonstick spray and spread a few spoonful of sauce around in the bottom of the pan. Arrange 3 noodles, top with about 1 cup sauce, 1 cup creamy spinach mixture, and 3/4

cup Mozzarella cheese. Repeat for three complete layers. Top it all off with the last three lasagna noodles, 1 cup sauce, and 1 cup Mozzarella cheese. Cover with greased foil so the cheese doesn't stick and bake for 40 minutes.

• Remove foil and bake for another 10 to brown the cheese (or turn on your broiler to get it browned). Remove from oven and let stand for 15 minutes before slicing and serving.

Cheesy Garlic Parmesan Spinach Spaghetti Squash

This crazy delicious garlic parmesan spaghetti s�uash is one of the most popular recipes on Peas and Crayons — and for good reason too!

Ingredients

- 1 medium spaghetti squash (approx. 2-3lbs)
- 2.5 TBSP minced garlic
- 1 tsp avocado oil or olive oil
- 5 oz fresh spinach chopped
- 1/2 cup heavy cream
- 1 TBSP cream cheese (optional but delicious!)
- 1/2 cup freshly grated parmesan cheese plus extra for topping
- salt and pepper to taste
- grated or sliced mozzarella for topping to taste

Instructions

• Pre-heat oven to 400 degrees F. Slice your spaghetti s⍰uash in half lengthwise and scoop out the seeds.

• For easy cutting, feel free to stick your s⍰uash in the microwave to soften it up just a tad. Pierce it a few times with a knife (to help vent so it doesn't burst) and cook for for 3-5 minutes. The knife slides through way easier this way! Smaller s⍰uash will need about 3 minutes while larger ones will be good to go at 4-5 min.

• Next grab a lipped baking sheet or a rimmed baking dish. Rub the cut side of the s⍰uash with a teeny bit of olive oil and place on your baking dish/sheet cut side down. Roast for about 40 minutes, or until tender and easily pierced with a fork. Cooking time will vary a bit depending on the size of your s⍰uash, and larger s⍰uash will need to roast a bit longer to tenderize. Once ready, the once rock-hard exterior of the s⍰uash will be visibly softened with a tender interior.

• The s⍰uash can be roasted and stored in the fridge for a few days if you'd like to meal prep and plan ahead for a speedier dinner. While the squash roasts, start on the sauce.

• In a medium pot or skillet, bring a drizzle of olive oil to medium-high heat and sauté garlic until fragrant. Next add the spinach and stir until wilted. Add your cream, cream cheese (totally optional but totally tasty) and parmesan cheese and stir well.

• Season with salt and pepper to taste and remove from heat. Once s�uash is done roasting, allow to cool until easily handled or pop on an oven mit and use a fork to separate and fluff the strands of spaghetti squash.

• Pour your sauce over each s�uash boat, stir to mix, and top with a little mozzarella cheese and additional parm cheese, if desired. Bake at 350 degrees F for around 20 minutes or until hot and bubbly. For a golden cheesy topping, flip your oven to broil on high for just a minute or two until lightly browned. Dive in while it's HOT!

Slow cooker potato soup

This hearty and healthy, super creamy potato soup recipe cooks up in your slow-cooker for hands-off cooking and delicious soup that will be ready for you when you get home from work.

Ingredients

- 1 (26 to 30-ounce) bag frozen hash browns
- 2 (14-ounce) cans non-fat chicken broth
- 1 (10.75-ounce) can 98% fat-free cream of chicken soup
- 1/4 cup onion, chopped
- 1/4 teaspoon black pepper
- 1 (8-ounce) package low-fat
- cream cheese
- 1 cup fat-free milk
- Green onions, chopped, to garnish
- Bacon bits, optional, to garnish

Instructions

Add hash browns, chicken broth, chicken soup, onion, and black pepper to your slow-cooker and cook on high for an hour. Stir, then turn your slow-cooker to low for another hour.

Add cream cheese, and cook another 1/2 hour or until cheese can be stirred into the mixture.

Add milk and cook 10 to 15 minutes longer.

Garnish with chopped green onion and bacon bits. Add 1 WW point for garnish.

Chicken & Tomato–Stuffed Spaghetti S�uash

Ingredients

• 1 large spaghetti s�uash

• salt, to taste

• pepper, to taste

• olive oil

• 2 boneless, skinless chicken breasts, cubed

• 3 cloves garlic, minced

• 4 roma tomatoes, diced

• 8 oz spinach (225 g)

• 24 oz marinara sauce (680 g), 1 jar

• ½ cup fresh basil (20 g)

• ¼ teaspoon red pepper, crushed

Instructions

1. Preheat oven to 375˚F (190˚C).

2. With a sharp knife, slice the s⍰uash in half. (If the s⍰uash is too tough - puncture in several places forming a dotted line around the s⍰uash. Microwave 3-5 minutes to soften. Allow to cool before cutting in half - following the dotted line).

3. Scoop out the seeds, brush with oil, salt, and pepper, and place face down on a baking tray. Bake for 35-40 minutes or until a fork can easily pierce the skin.

4. Heat olive oil in a large pan. Add chicken breasts (seasoned with salt and pepper) and garlic, and fully cook.

5. Add tomatoes and spinach. Cook until spinach has wilted. Add marinara sauce.

6. Stack the basil leaves and roll them up. Cut into slices and add to pan.

7. Add crushed red pepper, and stir until the ingredients are fully incorporated.

8. Once the s⍰uash has finished roasting, remove from the oven and let it sit for a few minutes before turning over and pulling at it with a fork. (Careful, there will be some steam!)

9. Shred the inside of each s�uash, being careful not to poke through the skin. Pour the sauce over the shredded s�uash, top with fresh basil, and serve.

10. Enjoy!

Quinoa Black Bean Crockpot Stuffed Peppers

These Quinoa Black Bean Crockpot Stuffed Peppers can be made with or without meat – all with simple pantry ingredients! Minimal prep, awesome taste.

Ingredients

- 6 bell peppers
- 1 cup uncooked ▯uinoa, rinsed
- 1 14 ounce can black beans, rinsed and drained
- 1 14 ounce can refried beans
- 1 1/2 cups red enchilada sauce
- 1 teaspoon cumin
- 1 teaspoon chili powder
- 1 teaspoon onion powder
- 1/2 teaspoon garlic salt
- 1 1/2 cups shredded Pepperjack cheese
- toppings! cilantro, avocado, sour cream, etc.

Instructions

1. Cut the tops off of the peppers and scrape out the ribs and seeds.

2. In a large bowl, combine the ⍰uinoa, beans, enchilada sauce, spices, and 1 cup of the cheese. Fill each pepper with the ⍰uinoa mixture.

3. Pour 1/2 cup water into the bottom of a crockpot. Place the peppers in the crockpot so they're sitting in the water. Cover and cook on low for 6 hours or high for 3 hours. Remove lid, distribute remaining cheese over the tops of the peppers, and cover again for a few minutes to melt the cheese.

4. Serve topped with anything you like! These are also great with chips and guacamole, believe it or not.

Crock Pot Salmon With Lemon and Herbs

Ingredients

• 1 to 2 pounds skin-on salmon fillets

• Salt

• Fresh ground black pepper

• Spices (optional)

• Sliced lemon (optional)

• Sliced aromatic vegetables, like fennel, onions, or celery (optional)

• 1 to 1 1/2 cups liquid, such as water, broth, wine, beer, cider, or a mix

Instructions

1. Cut the salmon into pieces. I usually cut the salmon into large pieces roughly the same size of my slow cooker, placing the smaller piece on top of the larger one. You can also cut them into smaller, individual-serving fillets.

2. Sprinkle salmon with salt and pepper. Season the flesh side of the salmon with salt and pepper. Be generous!

Sprinkle on any other spices you're using and rub them in with your fingers.

3. Line the slow cooker. Cut a large square of parchment or aluminum foil and press it into the slow cooker. This makes it easier to lift the delicate salmon out of the slow cooker later.

4. Place aromatics over the bottom of the slow cooker. If you're using them, place a layer of lemon slices and sliced aromatics on the bottom of the slow cooker. This adds flavor, but isn't strictly necessary.

5. Place one layer of salmon in the slow cooker. Place the larger piece of salmon skin-side down in the slow cooker. Top with more slices of lemon and aromatics, if using.

6. Add another layer, if needed. If you're cooking more salmon than fits in a single layer, you can add a second layer. Place a piece of parchment or foil over the first layer, lay the rest of the salmon over skin-side down, and top with aromatics. (I don't recommend adding a third layer.)

7. Choose your cooking liquid. The li�uid helps to poach the salmon gently. It can be as simple as plain water, or as

complex as a cup of amber beer with soy sauce and fish sauce mixed in. My standby is half water and half white wine. You'll need between 1 and 1 1/2 cups of li�uid.

8. Pour the li�uid over the salmon. If cooking one layer, add enough li�uid to just barely cover. If cooking two layers, add enough li�uid to come partway up the side of the top fillet.

9. Cook on LOW for 1 to 2 hours. Cover and cook on the LOW setting. The exact cooking time will vary based on your particular slow cooker, the number and thickness of your fillets, and how "done" you like your salmon. Check the salmon after 1 hour and continue checking every 20 minutes until it's done. If you prefer fully cooked salmon, check it with a thermometer in the thickest part — the fish is done when it reaches 145°F.

10. Remove from the slow cooker. Lift the salmon from the slow cooker by grasping the parchment or aluminum foil. Tilt the paper slightly as you lift to drain off the li�uid. Serve immediately, or cool and refrigerate.

Chicken, Potatoes, and Green Beans

This one-pot Slow Cooker Seasoned Chicken, Potatoes and Green beans has a homemade dressing/marinade and will be your new favorite healthy dinner.

Ingredients:

• 2 lbs. Boneless Skinless Chicken Breasts

• 1/2 lb. fresh green beans trimmed (about 2.5 cups)

• 1 1/4 lb. diced red potatoes about 4 cups

Homemade dressing ingredients:

• 1/3 cup FRESH lemon juice (NOT BOTTLED) (1 large or 2 small lemons)

• 1/4 cup olive oil

• 1 tsp. dried oregano

• 1 tsp. salt

• 1/4 tsp. pepper

• 1/4 tsp. onion powder

• 2 garlic cloves minced

Instructions:

• Start by placing the chicken the middle of the slow cooker. Next, add the green beans on one side. Then for the potatoes, you will need to mound them high off to the other side. In a medium-sized bowl, whisk together the lemon juice, olive oil, oregano, salt, pepper, onion powder, and garlic cloves.

• Pour this mixture evenly over the chicken, green beans and potatoes. Cover and cook on HIGH for 4 hours or LOW for 7 hours, without opening the lid during the cooking time.

Slow Cooker Black Bean Butternut Chili

This make-ahead slow cooker black bean butternut chili is perfect nutritious vegan comfort food. Made with protein rich beans and ⍰uinoa as well as filling butternut s⍰uash. It's a perfect recipe for your weekly meal prep, and it freezes well!

Ingredients

For the chili:

- 2 teaspoons olive oil
- 1 large white or yellow onion, diced
- 2 stalks celery, diced
- 3 cloves garlic, minced
- 2 tablespoons tomato paste
- 1 1/2 tablespoons chipotle en adobo (about 1 pepper with juices, chopped)
- 2 teaspoons chili powder
- 1 teaspoon cumin
- 1 teaspoon coriander

• 1/2 teaspoon smoked paprika

• 1/2 teaspoon cinnamon

• 3/4 teaspoon salt, or to taste

• Pinch cayenne pepper, to taste

• 3 cups low sodium vegetable broth or water

• 3 cups cooked black beans (2 14.5-ounce cans, drained and rinsed)

• 1 – 1 1/4 pounds peeled and cubed butternut s⍰uash (about 1 small s⍰uash)

• 1 1/2 cups fire-roasted, diced tomatoes with their juices (1 14.5-ounce can)

• 1 cup dry ⍰uinoa

• Optional toppings: Tofu sour cream below, chopped green or red onions, chopped parsley, chopped cilantro, avocado slices, guacamole, hot sauce

For the tofu sour cream:

• 8 ounces silken tofu

• 2 teaspoons olive oil

• 2 tablespoons lime juice

• 2 teaspoons rice vinegar or white wine vinegar

• 3/4 teaspoon salt

Instructions

1. To make the tofu sour cream, simply place all ingredients in a blender or a food processor and blend till smooth.

2. Rinse the ⍰uinoa through a fine sieve under cold, running water. Allow it to drain while you proceed with the recipe.

3. For the most flavorful chili results, heat the olive oil in a large sauté pan over medium heat. Add the onions and celery and a pinch of salt, to get the onions sweating. Sauté for about 5 minutes, or until the onions are soft and clear. Add the garlic and cook for about 1 minute, stirring frequently. Add 1/4 cup water, the tomato paste, the chipotle en adobo, the chili powder, cumin, coriander, smoked paprika, cinnamon, salt, and cayenne. Allow it to cook for one more minute, stirring to incorporate all of the ingredients.

4. Add the broth, black beans, squash, diced tomatoes and their juices, and quinoa to your slow cooker. Add the cooked onion, garlic, and spice mixture. Stir everything to combine well. Cook on low heat for 6 hours. Before serving, give the chili a good stir and add some additional vegetable broth if you'd like it to be less thick. Taste, adjust seasonings, and serve with toppings of choice.

5. Alternately, you can simply add all of the ingredients to the slow cooker and cook for 6 hours on low. If you have the time, browning the onions and garlic will give you most flavor. See note for stovetop option!

Chicken Soup Slow Cooker

A one-pot chicken soup with a nourishing broth made from chicken bones, fresh thyme, garlic. Loaded with bright vegetables and tender, fall off the bone chicken.

Ingredients

- 2 lb Chicken Thighs (about 5 thighs)
- ½ Tbsp Real Salt
- ¼ tsp Pepper
- 2 Fresh Thyme
- 2 Cloves Garlic
- 5 Cups Chicken Stock
- 2 Tbsp Chicken Base (if using water instead of chicken broth)
- 1 lb Carrots (sliced in half lengthwise and cut into ¼" slices)
- 1 Yellow Onion
- ½ Bunch Kale (chopped into bite-sized pieces, about 4 cups packed)

• ½ Tbl Fresh Thyme

• To Taste Real Salt

Instructions

1. Place the chicken thighs in the base of a crock pot. Sprinkle the salt and pepper over the chicken. Place the thyme sprigs and minced garlic on top of the chicken.

2. Pour the water (or chicken broth) into the crock pot. Add the chicken base, if using. Cook the chicken on high for 4 hours. After 4 hours the chicken should be "fall off the bone" tender.

3. Remove the chicken from the crock pot and place in a bowl. Remove the thyme sprigs and discard. At this point, if you desire, you can strain the broth in the crock pot through a fine mesh sieve (if you want a broth free from any debris left from the chicken).

4. Add the broth back to the crock pot after straining. Turn heat back to high. Separate the chicken from the bones. Lightly shred the chicken. Discard any cartilage. Add the bones back to the soup and cover and refrigerate the chicken.

5. Add the carrots, onions, and chopped thyme to the broth and cook on high for 2 hours. In the last ½ hour of cooking, add the kale to the soup. After 2 hours the carrots should be soft and tender, along with the kale. Remove the bones from the soup and discard.

6. Check the seasonings and add more salt or pepper as necessary. Add the chicken to the soup and allow to reheat for about 10 minutes. Do not stir too much or the chicken will become over-shredded.

7. Serve

Crock Pot Beef and Broccoli

Tender beef and broccoli florets simmer in a slow cooker to create this warm and hearty Crock Pot Beef and Broccoli! It's a recipe that truly belongs in your dinner hall of fame!

Ingredients

• 2 pounds sirloin steak or boneless beef chuck roast sliced thin

• 1 cup beef broth

• 1/2 cup low sodium soy sauce

• 1/4 cup brown sugar

• 1 Tablespoon sesame oil

• 3 garlic cloves minced

• 4 Tablespoons cornstarch

• 4 Tablespoons water

• 1 bag (12 ounces) frozen broccoli florets

• cooked white rice to serve with (if desired)

Instructions

1. In the insert of a 6 quart crock pot (slow cooker), whisk together beef broth, soy sauce, brown sugar, sesame oil, and garlic.

2. Place slices of beef in the li�uid and toss to coat. Cover with lid and cook on low heat for 5 hours.

3. When beef is done cooking, whisk together cornstarch and water in small bowl. Pour into crock pot and stir to mix well.

Add the frozen broccoli over the beef and sauce. Gently stir to combine. Cover with lid and cook 30 minutes to cook broccoli and thicken sauce.

4. Serve over warm white rice. Enjoy!

Slow Cooker Asian Chicken Lettuce Wraps

These Slow Cooker Asian Chicken Lettuce Wraps are so simple to put together and make such a delicious and healthy weeknight dinner.

Ingredients

- 2 lbs ground chicken (not ground chicken breast)
- 3 cloves garlic , minced
- 1 red bell pepper , cored and finely chopped
- 1/2 cup finely chopped yellow onion
- 1/2 cup hoisin sauce
- 2 Tbsp soy sauce
- Salt and freshly ground black pepper
- 1 (8 oz) can sliced water chestnuts, drained and rinsed
- 1 1/2 cups cooked white or brown rice
- 3 green onions , sliced
- 1 Tbsp rice vinegar and 1 1/2 tsp sesame oil (optional)
- 2 heads iceberg lettuce

Instructions

1. Place ground chicken and garlic in a large microwave safe bowl. Microwave mixture, stirring occasionally, until chicken is no longer pink, about 5 - 6 minutes. Drain off li□uid and pour mixture into a 5 - 7 □uart slow cooker.

2. Add bell pepper, onion, hoisin sauce, soy sauce, 1/2 tsp salt and 1/2 tsp pepper and toss mixture. Cover and cook on low heat 2 - 3 hours until chicken is tender.

3. Stir in water chestnuts, cooked rice, green onions, rice vinegar, and sesame oil, cook until heated through 3 - 5 minutes. Season with additional salt as desired. Separate iceberg lettuce leaves and serve with chicken filling.

Hawaiian Pork Burrito Bowls

Slow Cooker Hawaiian Pork Burrito Bowls are a dinner saver as they cook all day in a homemade enchilada sauce then topped with sautéed peppers and juicy, seared pineapple!

Ingredients

Enchilada Sauce:

- (14.5 oz) can tomato sauce
- 2 tablespoon tomato paste
- 2 tablespoon chili powder
- 2 tablespoon cumin
- 1 teaspoon onion powder
- 1 teaspoon garlic powder
- 1/4 teaspoon paprika
- 1/8 teaspoon cayenne
- 1/4 teaspoon salt
- 1/4 teaspoon pepper

• 1 cup pineapple juice

Pork:

• 1 tablespoon coconut oil (or olive oil)

• 2 lbs pork sirloin roast

• 2 teaspoon cumin

• 1 teaspoon chile powder

• 2 teaspoon salt

• 2 teaspoon pepper

Garnish:

• 1/2 tablespoon coconut oil

• 1 1/2 cups □uinoa, uncooked, rinsed and drained

• 3 cups water

• 2 bell peppers, thinly sliced (I used red and orange)

• 1 green onion, thinly sliced

• 1 Pineapple, sliced into rings

• Avocado, sliced

• Cilantro, chopped

Instructions

Enchilada Sauce:

1. In a crock pot, add the ingredients for the enchilada sauce: tomato sauce through the pineapple juice. Whisk until well combined.

For the Pork:

2. In a large skillet, add the coconut oil and heat over medium high heat.

3. Season all sides of the pork with the cumin, chile powder, salt and pepper.

4. Add the pork to the skillet and sear on all sides, about 2 mins per side. Once seared add to a slow cooker. Spoon some of the enchilada sauce over the top of the pork. Cook on high for 3 1/2 hours, or until done.

5. Remove the pork from the slow cooker and onto a large plate. Shred with two forks. Place back into slow cooker and mix well with the sauce.

To serve:

6. Cook the quinoa according to the packages instructions. Set aside until ready to serve. Remove from the heat.

7. Meanwhile, in a large skillet, heat the coconut oil over medium heat. Add the peppers and sauté for 5 minutes or until soft. Remove from the heat and add the pineapple slices. Cook until slightly browned, about 1 minute.

8. To serve, add quinoa to a bowl, top with the pepper mixture then the pork. Garnish with the pineapple rings, avocado and cilantro.

Honey Garlic Shredded Beef Tacos

With fall-apart tender honey garlic beef, roasted vegetables and crumbled feta cheese, these shredded beef tacos are a huge hit! Simple to prepare and can be meal prepped.

Ingredients

Roasted Vegetables

- 2 zucchinis cubed; roughly 4 cups
- 2 bell peppers chopped into ½ inch cubes
- ½ red onion cut into chunks
- ½ tablespoon olive oil
- salt and pepper
- 1 cup cherry tomatoes halved

Tacos

- 8 small tortillas
- 2 cups Slow Cooker Honey Garlic Beef
- ½ cup feta cheese crumbled

• 1 lemon cut into wedges

• yogurt or tzatziki to serve

Instructions

Roasted Vegetables

• Pre-heat oven to 400°F. Toss the zucchini, bell pepper and red onions in the olive oil. Place in a baking dish. Sprinkle with salt and pepper. Roast for 15 minutes. Add the tomatoes to the dish and return to the oven for 5 more minutes.

To assemble a taco

• Place ¼ cup of pulled beef on a 6-inch tortilla. Top with roasted veggies. Sprinkle with feta, squeeze lemon over, and top with yogurt/tzatziki if desired

Crock Pot Spaghetti S⍰uash Thai 'Noodle' Bowl

This squash needs a full eight or nine hours in the Crock-Pot, so it's the perfect thing to leave on while you're at work all day. When you get home: Shred, sauce, and feast.

Ingredients:

• 1 Small Spaghetti Squash (About 4-5 lbs.

• 2 C. Water

• 2 C. Broccoli, Steamed

• 1/2 Batch Prepared Skinny Thai Peanut Dressing (I used Lime Juice instead of 1/2 of the Vinegar for mine.)

• 1 Tbsp. Sesame Seeds

Optional/Suggested Toppings:

• Chopped Peanut

• Sriracha

Directions

• Pierce your spaghetti s⍰uash all over with a fork (similarly to how you would with a potato before baking.)

• Place the s�uash and 2 c. of water into a slow cooker. Secure the lid and cook for 8-9 hours on low.

• Once done, remove the squash from the crock pot and set aside to cool for 20-30 minutes. Discard the water.

• After the s�uash has cooled, cut it in half and scoop out the seeds and pulp. It should all come out pretty easily. Mine even separated from the meat of the squash on it's own. Discard or use for something else if you want.

• With the pulp removed, use a fork to shred the insides into spaghetti like noodles.

• Place the 'noodles' into a bowl and top each with 1 c. of broccoli, 3 tbsp. dressing, 1/2 tbsp. sesame seeds, and peanuts if desired. Enjoy!

Slow cooker apricot chicken

A simple slow cooker apricot chicken that has big fresh flavors and an intoxicating aroma!

Ingredients

- 1 teaspoon extra virgin olive oil
- 2 lbs. boneless, skinless chicken thighs
- 1/2 teaspoon salt
- 1/4 teaspoon black pepper
- 1 cup low-sodium chicken broth
- Zest and juice of 1 lemon
- 3 tablespoons Dijon mustard
- 4 garlic cloves, minced
- 1 teaspoon dried thyme
- 1 cup sliced onion
- 1 cup dried apricots, halved if desired

Instructions

1. Heat olive oil over medium-high heat in a large saute pan.

2. Season chicken thighs with salt and pepper. Add to pan and cook for 5-6 minutes, until browned, turning once.

3. Combine chicken broth, lemon zest and juice, mustard, garlic and thyme in slow cooker and whisk to combine. (Or you can stir it all together in a small bowl and add to your slow cooker.)

4. Add onions, apricots and seared chicken thighs to the slow cooker.

5. Cover and cook on low for 6-8 hours or high for 3-4 hours.

6. Serve chicken thighs and plenty of sauce over brown rice or whole wheat couscous.

CONCLUSION

Gout is no longer a disease of rich monarchs who overindulge in fatty meats and wine, but a health problem that can affect anyone. Foods rich in purines can raise blood levels of uric acid. Deposits of urate can form crystals in the joints, resulting in gout's miserable inflammation and pain. Males, and people living with kidney problems, obesity, high blood pressure and high levels of fat in the blood are especially at risk.

In addition to medication, regular exercise, weight loss, ade�uate hydration and avoiding alcohol, meal planning with the right recipes can reduce levels of uric acid in the body – and the resulting painful crystal formation.

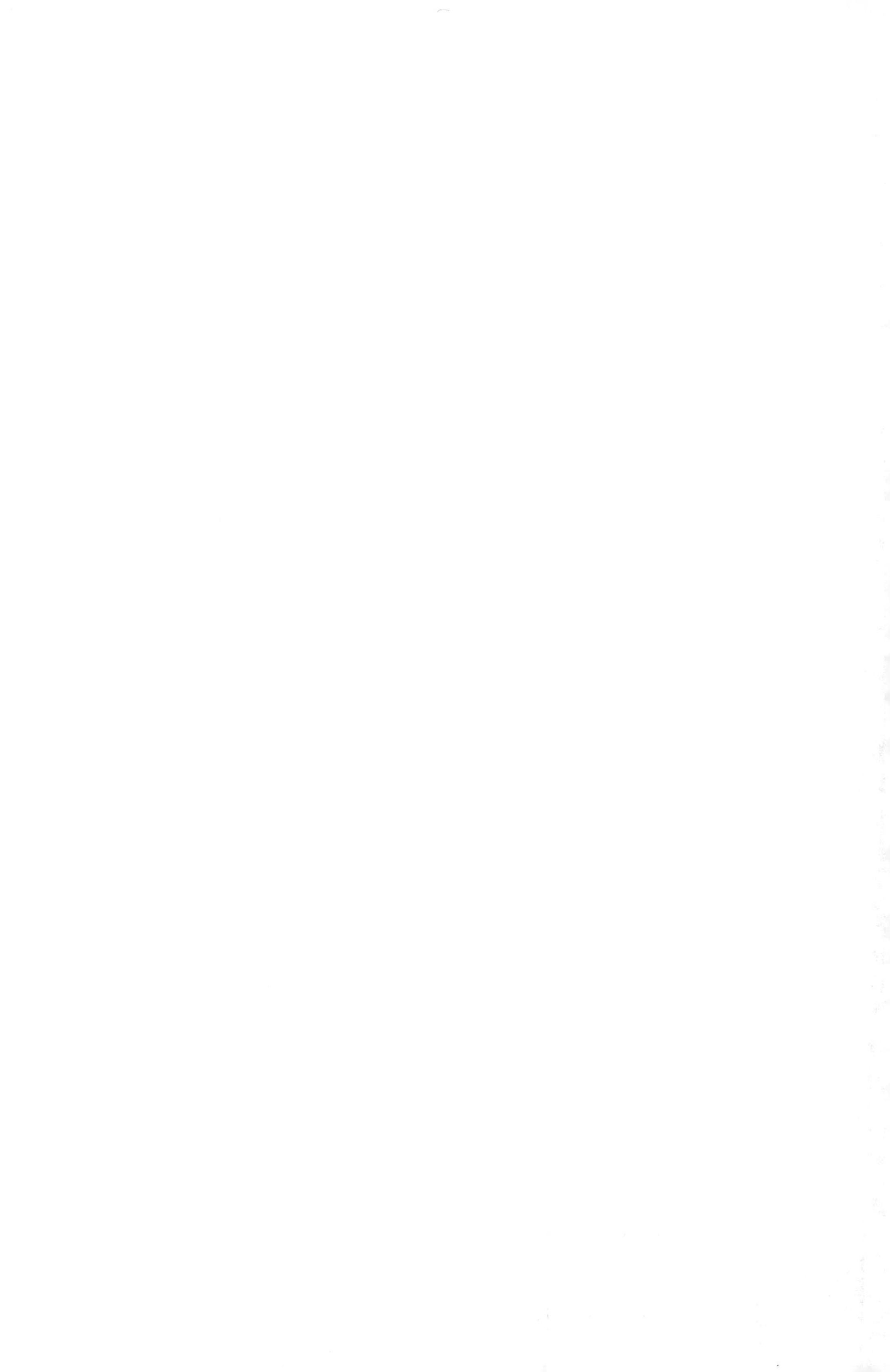

www.ingramcontent.com/pod-product-compliance
Lightning Source LLC
LaVergne TN
LVHW050316160826
845677LV00014B/3426

9798360830320